the perfect fit

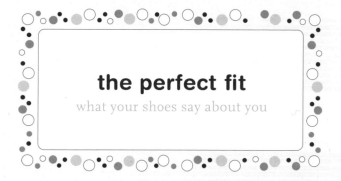

the perfect fit

what your shoes say about you

by meghan cleary
illustrations by sydney vandyke

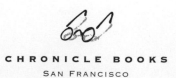

CHRONICLE BOOKS

SAN FRANCISCO

Library of Congress
Cataloging-in-
Publication Data
available.

ISBN 0-8118-4501-X

Manufactured in China.

Designed by Lesley Feldman,
Seattle, Washington

Distributed in Canada
by Raincoast Books
9050 Shaughnessy Street
Vancouver, British Columbia V6P 6E5

10 9 8 7 6 5 4 3 2 1

Chronicle Books LLC
85 Second Street
San Francisco, California 94105

www.chroniclebooks.com

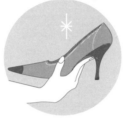

*To the women who
handed down their joy to me like a
bejeweled, couture-quality shoe:
Grandma, Mary, Mom*

My sweets, Miss Meghan here, expert sole searcher and
arch supporter. I hope you know how I love you and
adore you. And because I love you and adore you so, I
want you to understand the divine work of art that you
are. How? you may ask. Through the very objects that
house your sole, my dear: *your shoe.*

As you probably know, the shoe — more than any accessory
— defines the woman. And my purpose is to help you come
to a thorough and profound understanding of who you are
and what the future may hold, as evidenced by the shoes you
wear: discover the careers that best fit you, what to look for
in seeking a Sole Mate, and how to invoke your inner stiletto.
This charming and divinatory book you hold in your hands
is filled with the tools you'll need for all of the above.

First, turn to Chapter 1, wherein we'll identify your Shoe
Sun sign and your basic sole, and you'll explore the dark con-
tents of your wardrobe. Then in Chapters 2, 3, and 4 you'll
explore different shoe personalities and connect with the
ones that best define you. With that foundation, we will pro-
ceed to a deeper understanding of the complexities of your
sole: your Shoe Rising signs, touchstones that will guide you
to the right shoe choices in every situation, and your Shoe
Opposites, which will pinpoint fears, hesitations, and unex-
plored territory in your psyche.

Why sole-search, you may ask. Ever since Catherine de
Medici seductively undulated her way into the French court

in 1533, mesmerizing everyone in the room including her husband — the French king Henry II — the shoe has become a symbol of feminine beauty and desire. Whether you're a Stiletto with Barefoot Rising, or a Mary Jane with Sneaker Rising, you will learn to appreciate the raw feminine force of your own shoe sign and to expand your deepest knowledge of your self.

So with that, I urge you to read on, my dearies! It's going to be ever so fun.

Miss Roxy

WHAT EXACTLY IS A STILETTO?

The word "stiletto" originates from the lovely Latin word stylus, *meaning "slender dagger." Doesn't that just send naughty shivers up your spine? Believed to have been created for Catherine de Medici in the 1530s, stilettos had their rebirth in 1955 when Roger Vivier designed a pointy, high heel fortified with a thin metal heel tube for Dior. This meant that ladies could enjoy the swaying seductive walk stilettos offered, with minimum breakage; this was the precursor of the luscious stiletto we enjoy today, which has been made even more durable with the advent of plastic!*

It is said that the shape of a woman's foot in a stiletto mimics the shape of the leg and foot during extreme sexual arousal, which is a delicious little tidbit to think about. At the very least, a stiletto always gets you to strike a pose, however unconsciously, and turns you into the natural seductress you are.

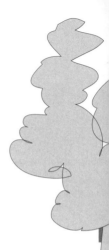

CHAPTER ONE

miss meghan asks: shoe *are* you?

Welcome to the first step in knowing the
real shoe you. Take the insightful quizzes inside
this chapter to discover your Shoe Sun sign,
Rising sign, Opposite sign, and even what the
shoes you *didn't* buy say about you!
Ready to peek inside your sole? Let's get
started, my sweets!

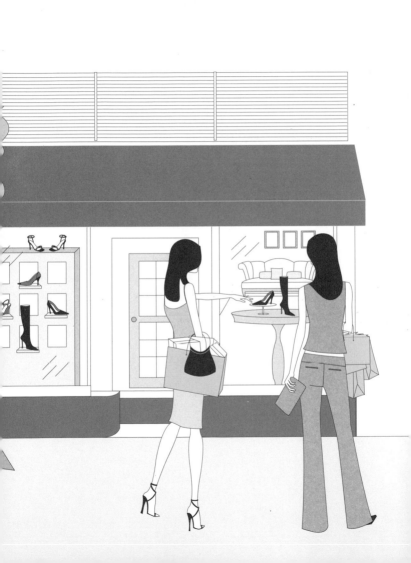

shoe *are* you?

Like star signs, shoe girls fall into basic categories: In this case, Down-to-Earth, On-the-Go, and Towering Heights. Chapters 2, 3, and 4 further define these types, as well as offer the related shoe signs and personality descriptors. But before any of this information can be truly useful, we must do a few, sole-searching exercises.

First, *shoe* are *you*?

1. What is your favorite pair of shoes?

....

2. List three adjectives that describe these shoes *(example: comfortable, expensive, drop-dead gorgeous).*

....

....

....

3. List three adjectives that describe how you feel when you wear these shoes *(example: I feel joyous, confident, sexy).*

....

....

....

4. List three compliments you've received from friends and admiring observers *(example: You sexy thing! Where did you find those? Your legs go on forever!).*

....

....

....

5. Flip through the next three chapters in the book to find the shoe that most closely matches your favorite shoe. Then write the shoe type here.

....

The shoe you've just identified is your Shoe Sun sign, your most natural state of being. The adjectives you've listed about the feelings you experience in these shoes are the attributes you exude when you are in your most confident and divine state of shoe. Your Shoe Sun sign is your true north, the place of balance and bliss you should always strive for. Measure any and all future purchases against this shoe sign.

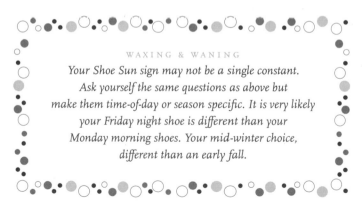

WAXING & WANING

Your Shoe Sun sign may not be a single constant.
Ask yourself the same questions as above but
make them time-of-day or season specific. It is very likely
your Friday night shoe is different than your
Monday morning shoes. Your mid-winter choice,
different than an early fall.

shoe do you want to be?

Now, Miss Meghan knows that women are complex creatures. Your Shoe Sun sign, while certainly the main character, is not the whole story. Searching your sole should never be so easy. Miss Meghan wants to know:

Shoe do you want to be?

1. What is the last pair of shoes you wanted to buy but didn't? Perhaps you went so far as to bring them home but later returned them in a fit of self-doubt?

....

2. Flip through the next three chapters to find the type of shoe that most closely matches the shoe you nearly bought. Then write the shoe type here. (Don't be surprised if it's a stiletto. Miss Meghan has found many women naturally incline toward their inner Stiletto.)

....

3. List three positive adjectives that describe these shoes *(example: comfy, hot, sleek)*.

....

....

....

4. List three negative adjectives that describe these shoes *(example: expensive, trendy, uncomfortable)*.

....

....

....

The shoe you've identified is your Shoe Rising sign, the state of shoe you aspire to. It's important to note that you may have several rising signs, so repeat the questionnaire as the mood strikes. The positive adjectives you list identify aspects of your sole that might need some added support. The negative adjectives identify fears about or barriers to achieving that support. Identifying your Shoe Rising sign is key to moving beyond where you are now and charting a path toward where you want to go.

moving beyond your fears

Review the three adjectives you wrote in response to question 4 in "*Shoe* do you want to be?" Now, see if any of those adjectives match these. Underneath each, you'll find some advice based on your resistance!

outrageous, scandalous, shocking
Try dramatic, spectacular, fabulous! *You are clearly suppressing an innate desire to wear stilettos to the office. Let go, girl! Give it a try!*

frivolous, childish, silly
Try whimsical! *You need more fun in your life. Leave what you are doing right now and run to the store where you saw them. Buy them, take them home, and put on an outfit worthy of these shoes! Flaunt your whimsy!*

expensive, extravagant
Clearly, it's time to assess what your happiness is worth. Why don't you feel you deserve these shoes?

strange, bizarre
How about unique? You picked them up for a reason. Unusual design, texture, or shape may be just what Miss Meghan would order for you. Is something not working for you exactly the way you'd like it to? Don these and stride into your life with the intent of making it work!

too high

Unless there is a medical reason for disdaining high heels, then don't. Perhaps this offers a little look-see into your unwillingness to tower. Don't be afraid of your own brilliance! Towering, if only occasionally, can enhance your natural female divinity.

too low

Are you are a high-heel junkie? Some time closer to the earth may be what you secretly crave. And don't worry, you're not selling yourself short. Feeling the earth move under your feet could be just the vibe you're looking for.

not designer

Uh-oh. Looks like a serious case of designer-itis. You've got to mix the high and low cultures to have fun, my friend.

bright, colorful

Baby, you need some diversity in your life. You may not find an everyday use for that pair of kelly-green python pumps or those purple suede stilettos, but that doesn't mean they don't belong.

opposites attract

Yes, there is such a thing as an Opposite Shoe sign. Find your Shoe Sun sign in the following chart. The shoe beside it is your Opposite Shoe sign. Opposites are a great tool for sole discovery, as they identify a path that deserves a little exploration and inner reflection. Do you consciously resist your Opposite? Do you have any friends who are Opposite? Read your Opposite's profile in Chapters 2, 3, or 4 and think seriously about what this says about you. Miss Meghan recommends you go so far as to seek out a pair of Opposites and wear them for at least a day. Before you judge, walk a mile in those shoes!

SHOE SUN SIGN	OPPOSITE SHOE SIGN
Barefoot	Designer Shoe
Flip-Flop	Ankle Boot with High Heel
Reef Sandal	Mule with High Heel
Classic Leather Thong Sandal	Pointy Toe Skimmer
Ballet Flat	Cowboy Boot
Designer Bowling Shoe	Classic Conservative Pump
T-Strap	Clog
Retro Basketball	Loafer

SHOE SUN SIGN	OPPOSITE SHOE SIGN
Mule, Flat	*Hiking Boot*
Running Shoe	*Open Toe*
High-Heel Sandal	*Clunky Chunky-Heel Loafer*
Stiletto	*Orthopedic Sandal*
Sneaker	*Knee-High Boot with High Heel*
Knee-High Boot with Low Heel	*Bedroom Slipper*
Mary Jane	*Workingman's Boot*

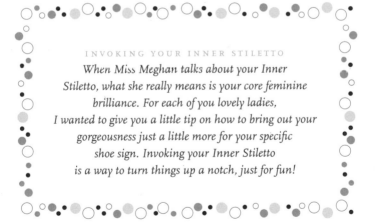

INVOKING YOUR INNER STILETTO

*When Miss Meghan talks about your Inner
Stiletto, what she really means is your core feminine
brilliance. For each of you lovely ladies,
I wanted to give you a little tip on how to bring out your
gorgeousness just a little more for your specific
shoe sign. Invoking your Inner Stiletto
is a way to turn things up a notch, just for fun!*

down-to-earth

The women who inhabit this basic sole type
like to feel grounded and in step with reality at all
times. The feel of the earth or pavement
beneath their feet gives them a feeling of stability
that helps them move through life with
a very consistent and steady pace, approaching all
situations with holistic understanding.
For these ladies, dressing up is more about letting
their inner beauty shine than about giving an
everyday show.

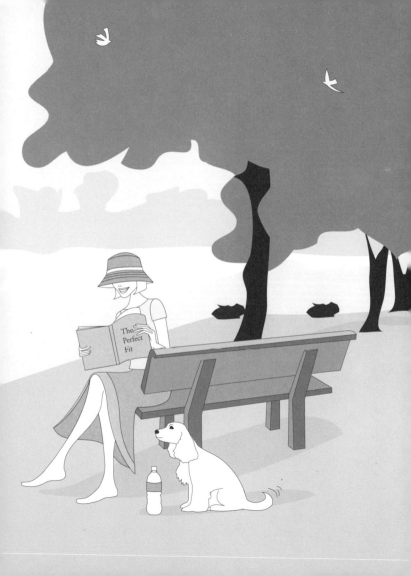

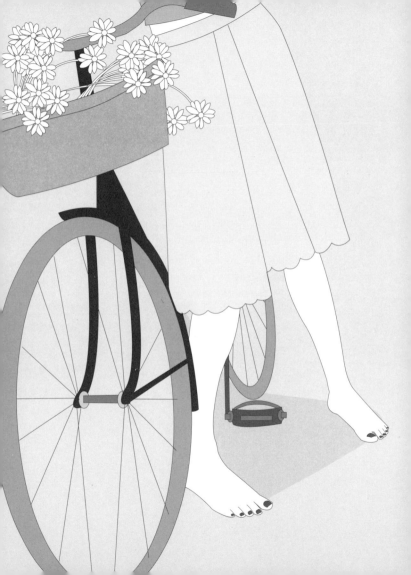

barefoot

You fancy yourself a naturalist, a hippie, or someone who just doesn't belong in shoes. Whatever your reason, you, the Barefoot girl, have eschewed shoes. You are eminently charming and lovable, carefree and breezy, and you usually add a breath of fresh air to any room you enter (sometimes along with a slight breeze of lavender-verbena aromatherapy).

You may have discovered your love of barefootedness in early childhood, when shoes restricted your natural independent spirit: you pleaded to go barefoot just another hour in the summer or into the fall, when most other children were slipping back into school shoes. Because your independence started early and is deeply ingrained in your sense of self, it is important that you are around those who value your free-spirited sensibility, for you can open their eyes to a whole new world.

Your friendships are formed with those who appreciate your grounded independence and correspond with more earth-centered issues like environmentalism and vegetarianism. However, you are very tolerant of all different walks of life. Since you yourself are considered a bit odd, you often befriend those who also need a bit of cheering from the outside world. A loyal friend, though sometimes hard to pin down, you will always be there, with many a natural remedy on hand, in any kind of crisis.

Traveling far and wide, you live in many different places, in search of new things to catch your eye and light up your idealism. Constant change is a fixed phenomenon in your lifestyle.

completing the look

Try breezy flowing skirts that do not hinder movement. Your hair, long and loose, looks nice tied up in a natural hemp ponytail holder, with tendrils slipping out. For makeup, try organic olive-oil soap and fresh aloe, and cherry-flavored lip gloss. Earrings are long and flowy and usually handmade (try the ones you picked up in that Southwestern town you lived in for a while) by a local artisan. Try wearing a few rings made out of natural fibers and sometimes an ankle bracelet or two, which tinkle quietly as you enter the room.

work it, girl

Go for what your heart leads you to, what is right instinctively both for you and for a larger cause. You'll work tirelessly, but you must be mentally engaged and a true believer in whatever task you take on. An occupation that gives you flexibility, freedom, and an unstructured environment is always preferred. Volunteering at the local food co-op or Habitat for Humanity, marching in a rally for peace, and working on voter registration are good projects. Varied tasks are key as boredom is a great danger for your spirit. Interacting with people and using your hands are also important.

While loving just as freely as you meander, you are not indiscriminate. Your loves are as heartfelt, sweet, and pure as that third-grade crush. You fall hard and are often disappointed for you have extremely high ideals when it comes to love. Learning to manage your expectations in order to be happy and fulfilled in love is a key challenge. Your mate must have ideals as high as yours when it comes to believing in the goodness of the world and being engaged in life at a visceral level. A mate with a bit of practicality might benefit you, a little yin for your yang.

invoking your inner stiletto

Try a touch of organic sandalwood essential oil behind your ears. Known to induce lust in even the most stoic of individuals, it's a great way for you to turn it up a notch.

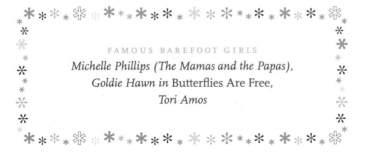

FAMOUS BAREFOOT GIRLS
Michelle Phillips (The Mamas and the Papas),
Goldie Hawn in Butterflies Are Free,
Tori Amos

bedroom slipper

You are a bit dreamy, half awake, half asleep. Your moniker is *cozy*. Often seen curled up on the couch in front of a daytime movie or just sipping your first cup of morning tea, you are surrounded by icons of comfort: flannel sheets, soft blankets, chocolate ice cream, lots of body lotion in lavender or green apple. Your movements are slow and languorous, with an innate sensuality you are almost unaware of but inhabit with the inner assurance of an eighteenth-century courtesan.

completing the look

Flannel or very soft well-worn cotton jersey-knit PJs are a must in pink, white, soft yellow, or mint green. Your hair is unwashed and often sticking up in some places, and makeup is clear lip balm and a rich face moisturizer. No jewelry and a slight natural rose flush colors the cheeks.

work it, girl

You are not *working* — you are *relaxing*.

finding a sole mate

Your mates are entranced by your dedication to comfort. You are the epitome of all earthly senses in their fully relaxed state. In order for your mates to understand you, they've got to get into the Zen vibe, too. You live in another world,

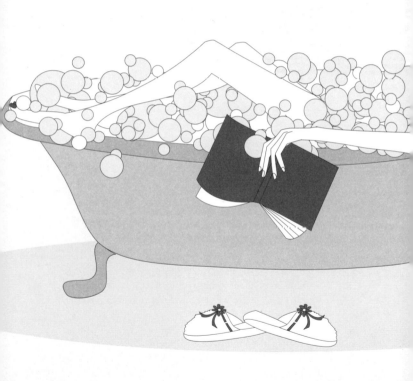

where things take time, and as soon as your mates understand this, they will be as relaxed and happy as you are.

invoking your inner stiletto

Slip into a transparent vintage nightie instead of your PJs — just as soft and sensual. Paired with your bedroom slippers, it's the best of high and low, sassy and sexy.

CUSTOM-MADE SHOES

A favorite topic of Miss Meghan's: custom-made, or couture, shoes. These of course are shoes made specifically for your feet only. Can you imagine! The sheer opulence of it. Trust me, it is truly divine. Typically, a shoemaker who specializes in custom work will take detailed measurements of your feet, let you select your style and materials, and voilà! Custom-made shoes feel like ecstatic slippers on your feet — they fit like a glove and since the materials are of an extremely high grade, they will mold to your feet as you wear them, creating a fit like no other. Pure luxury.

flip-flop

More often than not, you are on a boat or a dock. Very likely, you grew up on the water in a coastal town and know a sailboat like the back of your hand. Energetic and permanently tanned, you are a strong hand to have aboard any vessel. You can read a wave like a born surfer, and you like to race. Steady as a rudder, you are loyal and true to your good friends and in fact prefer their company après-sail to large social occasions. Having been in many a sea or Great Lake adventure, you sparkle with the energy of being truly alive, an intoxicating quality.

completing the look

Because you're so at home on the water, shorts and a tank top over a swimsuit become your natural elements of choice. Your hair, usually bleached a bit by the sun, can be thrown up in a messy ponytail or bun to keep it from interfering when you pull the jib. Since you've got an easy, natural beauty, the only makeup you need is sunscreen and a lip protectant.

work it, girl

You've got to be engaged with water to be happy, so marine biologist, whale-watch tour guide, dockhand, and competitive sailor are all good matches to keep your spirits up and your energy fluid.

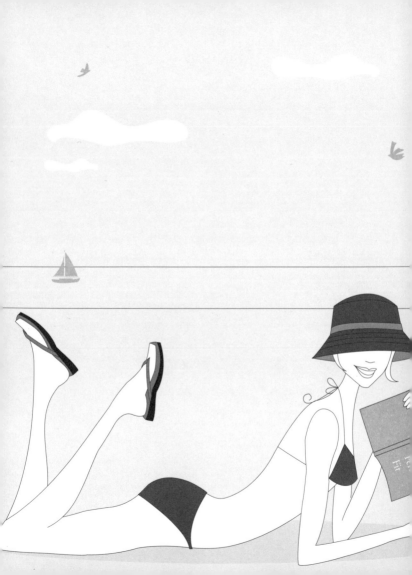

finding a sole mate

Your mate has got to love the water, obviously. In addition, you need to be with someone you admire, who secretly is your hero, whether because of coming in first in the America's Cup or knowing how to tie a knot with ease.

invoking your inner stiletto

Get fully SPF'd. Now pick out a bikini top that matches your eyes and pair it with your shorts, skipping the tank-top layering effect. Wonderful. I see the glow from here.

TO FLIP-FLOP OR NOT TO FLIP-FLOP

Flip-flops have become the center of some controversy as they have morphed from strictly poolside to all-occasion wear. While some women feel it perfectly acceptable to don a pair of flips with their suit when going to work in the summer (ew!), some, like Miss Meghan, find that choice downright offensive. Wherever you stand on the issue, there are exponential options to choose from, including flip-flops with a low kitten heel of molded rubber for a more dressy occasion or terry-covered flip-flops for a spa day.

reef sandal

You find yourself in reef sandals more than any other shoe and are therefore both sturdy and adventurous. You have many a trip to the Amazon and endangered tropical rain forests under your belt, and always ready for the next one, you radiate the energy of the perpetual traveler. You engineer modern public-health systems in developing countries as easily as you board the seaplane to your next destination. Unconcerned with material trappings, you believe that your next meal, house, or clothing will manifest itself without too much worry.

completing the look

Step out in easy, flexible pieces that wash well in any kind of water. All-natural cotton and moisture-wicking fabrics are important, in colors that are spirited: turquoise, purples, printed white tees, and tank tops. A swimsuit not only is for swimming but also is an integral extra layer, so multiple mix-and-match suits with durable construction are important. To easily camouflage the effect of limited showers, hair should be kept long. Makeup in the form of sunscreen and lip gloss complete the look.

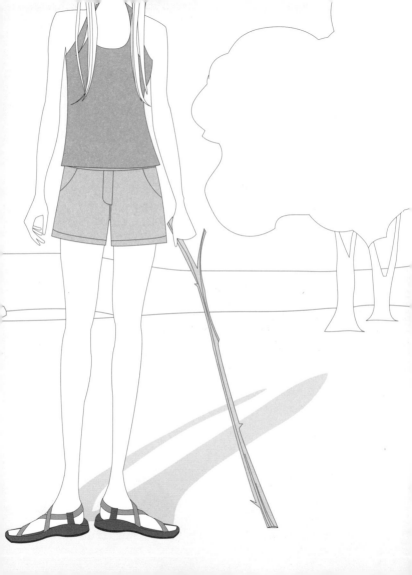

Ecotour leader. Your flair for adventure and your keen mind lead you to professions in which both intimate knowledge of geography and skill in traveling over rugged terrain are important. White-water rafting expeditions and rain-forest adventures are also great opportunities for you to apply your skills.

finding a sole mate

You need to be with a fellow adventurer, one who can bivouac with you through the mountainous terrain of life: a mate who is taken with natural beauty, has the unflagging spirit of a pioneer, and is physically hardy. A sense of humor is key so that you can laugh together at the latest Amazonian downpour from inside your tent.

invoking your inner stiletto

You're in the tropical rain forest, which is quite like a sauna. For your next adventure, try a polka-dot bikini, keep your sandals, and toss the rest into the jungle.

orthopedic sandal

Often startlingly beautiful, your glowing complexion may be the first thing that strikes a person upon meeting you. Because you are probably a vegan, the fruits and veggies you consume every day give you a natural, radiant glow. To the unenlightened, you may come across as complacent, but you shouldn't be underestimated: it's not that you are oblivious to the world around you; it's just that you see everything a little differently. Where one might see barren trees, you see stark beauty. Where one might see a thunderstorm, you see proof of nature's grace. Get the picture? Because of your ethereal nature, you are calming to be around. Though it may be an adjustment for those in your company to slow down enough to hang with you, they will find it well worth their while as you transmit to them a bit of your everyday joy — quite a nice feeling.

completing the look

Try flowered, flowing skirts, easy drawstring pants in a solid cotton, a soft tank top or oversize man's button-down shirt, knotted at the waist or thrown over your ensemble. Denim overalls and a wife beater are an easy way to inhabit your oeuvre as well. Hair is long or a chin-length bob, often pulled back in a headband or ponytail. Flavored lip gloss in a variety of all-natural fruity scents is all the makeup you need.

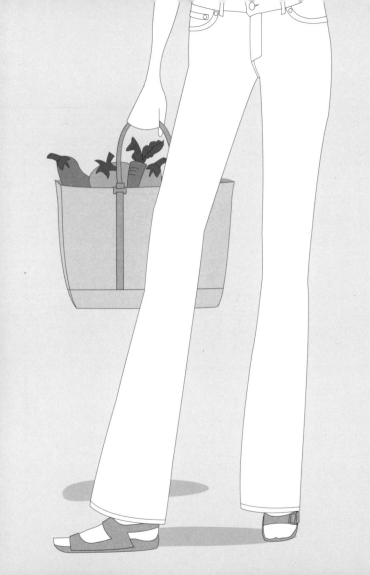

You are quite relaxed when it comes to working, always believing that things will work themselves out organically. Occupations in which you can engage with the natural world are recommended, be it a health-food co-op, a gardening gig, exterior housepainting, forestry or environmental work, or even involvement with Greenpeace. Since you may be a bit of the hidden artist, working on large outdoor sculpture, or painting nature landscape, would be beneficial. Rat-race 9-to-5 jobs are not recommended — they will kill your spirit in moments.

finding a sole mate

Your mate has to be as dedicated to unstructured living as you are: someone with solid values, who's well read, extremely understanding, and a bit quiet, though a mate who can really make your inner sweet giggle emerge is valuable, too. For that reason, playfulness is key in your equation of love.

invoking your inner stiletto

Oh, sweetie, let's lay the sandals aside for a moment and go barefoot, *non*? A little oil of sandalwood, perhaps? (See Barefoot, page 23.)

classic leather thong sandal

You take a resort attitude to life. Your pace is unhurried island time, a slower, more meditative approach. If it doesn't get done today, it can always get done tomorrow, or next week, for that matter. While others may get temporarily frustrated at your seeming lack of regard for their pace of life, they should actually be thankful, for you are the embodiment of the natural rhythm we should all strive for.

completing the look

Complete your look with a long casual skirt of cotton or linen and a tank top. Cotton shorts or clam diggers with a form-fitting tee in solid colors is a nice ensemble for you as well. Accessorize with a wide-brimmed straw hat and a bright tote for daily shopping. Your hair, short or long, is cut in layers and flowing or up in a casual bun. Makeup is a sheer pink lip gloss and a subtle glow in the cheek.

work it, girl

You've got to be in a flexible profession that allows you to enjoy open and airy spaces. A massage therapist or Pilates teacher at a luxury spa in an exotic locale, a high-fashion model on location, a photographer for a travel magazine, or even the owner of the local surf shop: all fit you well.

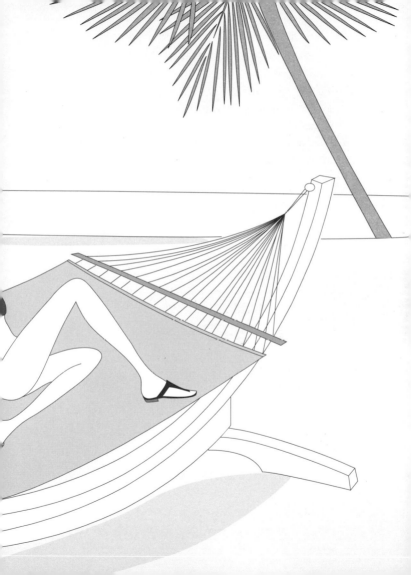

finding a sole mate

Look for a mate who embodies the attitude of a surfer (if not one already!). Someone who appreciates a slower pace, interested in the innate beauty and organic rhythm of life. Your mate should be able to laugh at absurdity just as easily as swinging into downward dog next to you on the yoga mat. Physically sturdy and fit, you and your mate should have a healthy dose of respect for each other.

invoking your inner stiletto

How about trying a short pleated skirt, plaiting your hair into lovely braids, and tucking a few fresh flowers behind your ears? Some dangling coral earrings, and you are really starting to shine.

ACCESSORIZE ME!

Your shoes need accessories, too. Satin ribbons, clip-on jewels, feather puffs, ostrich plumes, a delicate chain or two, even silk handmade flowers. Any of these are easy to find and quickly take it up a notch or two. Or three. (Even Hiking Boot girl can change her laces to purple, non?)

mule, flat

You are a real go-getter. Zipping around a party, town, or workplace, you all have one thing in common: your ability to look completely feminine and alluring without the addition of a high heel. You know that from the back you look like you've got nothing on your feet at all, and that a glimpse of bare heel can be sometimes sexier than a towering stiletto. Your close proximity to the ground means you know the trends early. A loyal friend, you've always got a bit of mischief up your sleeve, and without heels to slow you down, you are the one who is always first to the punch line.

completing the look

To get into a flat-heeled mule look, donning a somewhat funky outfit is required. A dress-over-pants ensemble is always a good foundation: tailored jeans with a cotton or cashmere jersey dress in a solid color that hits just above the knee is good for daytime. For evening, I see you in a ruched gauzy chiffon number of the same silhouette as daytime's over shiny satin cigarette pants, or a to-the-floor skirt of taffeta with a simple tight cashmere cardigan. Your hair should be down and flowing, and try a few key jewels — like a chunky ruby ring — to round out your look nicely.

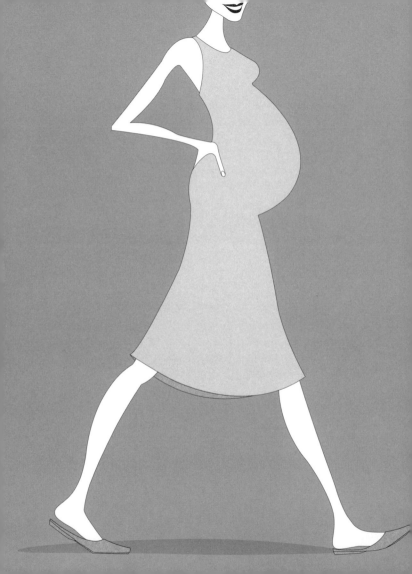

Your artistic edge, blended with your down-to-earth practicality, gives you a leg up at a photography studio, a graphic design firm, or a film production company. Anywhere creativity is housed and production is the goal, you will excel to no end.

finding a sole mate

You've got to be with someone who you can really let your hair down with. Life is a dance floor, and you like to get your groove on, so your mate has got to be willing to shake some booty with you. A mate who appreciates the arts or is an artist is key. Musicians are an excellent match for you, since you bring a little bit o' structure into their life while being sensitive to their artistic temperament.

invoking your inner stiletto

How about making that dress thrown over your jeans strapless — and pair it with a well-constructed push-up bra? A lacy, racy magenta shelf bra under your silk cardigan could be lovely, the buttons straining ever so slightly, with a tiny peek of that lacy stuff showing off your creamy flesh.

ballet flat

With a classic streak running though your veins, you either grew up in round-toe ballet flats or recently discovered some in your mother's closet while searching for vintage finds. For all your penchant for funky vintage looks, you are a daddy's girl, brought up with strong middle-class values. You excelled at school, but not in any brainiac kind of way, mostly because you worked hard and were polite to all of your teachers and kind to your classmates. Very often the class president, encouraged to run by your fellow classmates more than by any burning desire to be a political leader, you always had a steady boyfriend, a guy who was just as upstanding as you, and just as nice. You're the one who irons out disagreements between friends, sometimes without their even knowing it, and always with a lot of love. You are the core of any group of girlfriends, and as sweet as you are, you've been known to pull an outrageous prank or two when the conditions were ripe!

completing the look

Pair your ballet flats with a tailored designer jean. A solid-color very soft tee and a jacket that is figure-flattering and extremely feminine, often with a floppy silk flower pin on the lapel, completes the look. Makeup is simple and clean, tinted moisturizer so natural you just appear to have flawless

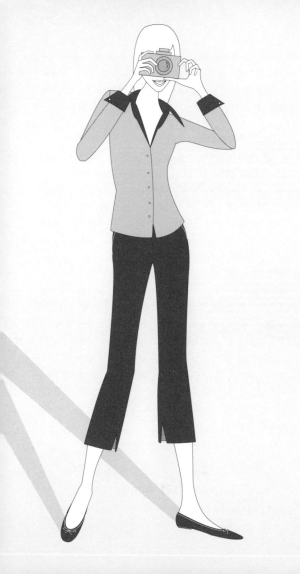

skin and that rosy glow. Jewelry is diamond studs. For evening, don a pair of sparkly ballet flats and a sparkly top to match; still in the jeans, you'll give a look of elegance and modernity at the same time.

work it, girl

You like a bit of structure in your life, even if you're at a funky downtown design firm. For that reason, an office environment appeals to you. Try fields in which your ethics will shine and your creativity can be nurtured. A nonprofit working on behalf of the less fortunate, children, or art is a good place to land. Private companies in fashion, graphic, or interior design that give back to the community are also recommended.

finding a sole mate

A mate who can put you at ease is crucial. Someone who is confident, a bit teasing, and funny at the same time is perfect, as you appreciate teasing as a sign of affection. You need to be with mates who are worthy of your time and attention and will make you proud to stand next to them. Above average in looks, your mate needs to adore you profoundly for you to feel happy.

invoking your inner stiletto

Lacy. Lacy. Lacy. Camisole, bra, panties, earrings. Voilà!

pointy toe skimmer

Oh, you are smart, aren't you? And pert, too. Whipping around the office, making sure all p's and q's are taken care of. You might be getting your boss's coffee, with your pad of To Do's in hand, crossing each one off in perfect harmony with your rhythmic morning office survey, or making sure your desk drawers are in perfect order. The absolutely charming thing about you is that however together you might appear, you've always got a little something tripping up your image. Getting your skirt stuck on a file cabinet while you are diligently filing, falling off your chair unexpectedly in the middle of a dinner date, tripping into your boss's arms in the elevator. Rather than being entirely flummoxed, you manage it with a sweet innocent charm, always pausing to tuck your hair back behind your ear after each incident and going back to whatever task is at hand, with studied determination.

completing the look

Easy A-line skirts in a viscose/cotton blend, structured blouses, and feminine jackets nipped at the waist are all good choices for you. A careful reference to the 1960s with a modern update and high-quality materials with a touch of luxury — think a mink-trimmed cardigan sweater, for

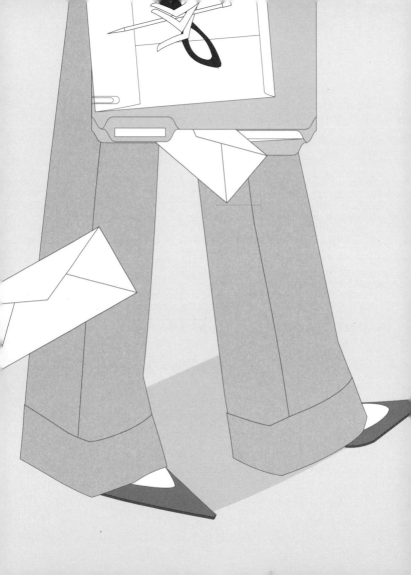

instance — further enhance your natural charms. Hair in a perky bob held back with a jeweled barrette and pink and red lipsticks always complement your look nicely.

work it, girl

You've got to be in an office. You are the one who adds a bit of glamour and style to the place as well as keeping it in thrumming and humming order, as if it ran by itself. Good fields to land in are real estate (you'd be the COO after working your way up from agent), a law firm (working your way to managing partner after being a legal assistant), and investment banking (you'd be the right-hand woman to the CEO).

finding a sole mate

With classic good looks and athletic and rugged in some ways, your mate has got to be a perfect blend of proper upbringing and unruffled attitude about your many careening episodes. In fact, your mate has to find your episodes completely and totally lovable — finding them the most charming thing about you!

invoking your inner stiletto

You know what? I think a black lace garter belt, sans panties, underneath your skirt will really have you feeling your femininity nicely.

mary jane

The Mary Jane girl's heart almost always harkens back to the era where girls were girls and boys were boys, and life ticked along with regularity. You like order and neatness in all things, though you are often game for a fun activity (provided it's not too outlandish) and have a great sense of playfulness underneath your prim and proper exterior. You may even pull the occasional complicated practical joke — extremely well orchestrated, of course. But that won't come until you know your victims quite well. You think the colors pale pink, yellow, and mint green are primary colors. Coordination is also a theme with you. In your mind, there is absolutely no reason that one's umbrella, trench coat, and rubber rain boots (I know you wear rubber rain boots on rainy days before you change into your Mary Janes indoors) shouldn't coordinate. Same with your kitchen — freshly lined kitchen shelves stocked with friendly, serviceable cups and saucers in coordinating colors are de rigueur. In your bedroom, English country is the mainstay: coordinated duvet, sheets, curtains, and rug. Fortunately, you have very good taste, so the overall effect of the coordinating is more cheery and comfy than overwhelming. Your belief is that there is no reason not to have a little coordination in one's life, a very calming effect.

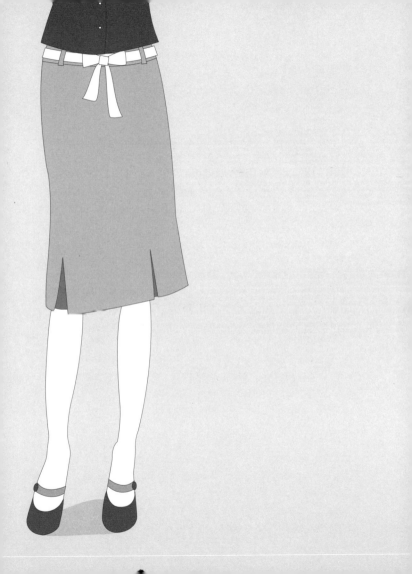

A freshly starched blouse and skirt ensemble always speaks to a Mary Jane girl. Quintessentially neat and crisply dressed, your jewelry should be pearls: coordinated necklace and earrings (given to you for your twelfth birthday by your mom) and an antique pearl ring from your grandma adorning your right pinkie finger. Hair swept back in a ponytail, often with a ribbon, and brushed at all times. Makeup is simple and traditional: lipstick in a color that matches a handbag or shoes, and neat, clean foundation with a touch of rose in the cheeks.

work it, girl

It is important that your skills are appreciated and you are given plenty of positive recognition. You will bloom and beam in these sorts of conditions. You will be happy using your detail skills at a local library, reorganizing the reference section, or working as an antique furniture restorer. As a high-powered executive assistant, successfully managing a very irascible boss with big business demands, your calm and soothing manner, along with your cool thinking and problem solving, would come into play.

finding a sole mate

A mate who opens doors and sends regular doses of fresh flowers (accompanied by a sweet note, of course) is the perfect match for you. Lawyers can be an excellent match as you appreciate their logic and rhetoric. And since they often find you the perfect companion, for you are perky, witty, and extremely considerate, this is a good combination. Other possible pairings include classical musicians, provided they are not too serious, and woodworkers.

invoking your inner stiletto

Donning a pair of racy, sheer boy-shorts underneath your skirt is the perfect way to harness your feminine wiles — they'll accentuate the plump roundness of your pink cheeks in a nice way that only you'll know about.

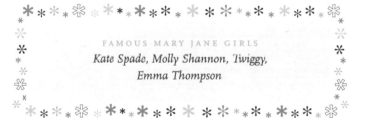

FAMOUS MARY JANE GIRLS
Kate Spade, Molly Shannon, Twiggy,
Emma Thompson

clog

The Clog girl moves with a feeling of solidity under her feet. No matter how hectic or chaotic things are, you are sure about where you are going and what you are going to attain. Your vibe is mellow, but don't mistake it for lazy. You are extremely hardworking and possess a deep spirituality, either consciously or unconsciously, which gives everything you do a sort of gravitas. Never giddy or overly excited, your natural state is an easy balance with not too many high highs or low lows.

completing the look

You'll be happiest in clothing you can move in; a printed flowing skirt or painters pants in khaki, denim, or faded dark red work well. Cotton boat-neck tees or tanks in neutral colors top off the outfit. Whatever the length, keep your hair off your face with a printed bandanna or simple hair tie, and keep the makeup to a minimum with a sheer peach lip gloss, just for enhancement, and a simple natural moisturizer for the face.

work it, girl

If you are a Clog girl, it is important for you to feel that you are contributing to the earth somehow in your work. A food co-op, an environmental outfit, a chef at an all-natural restaurant, and an organic farmer are all good ways to benefit the earth and work well with your natural groundedness.

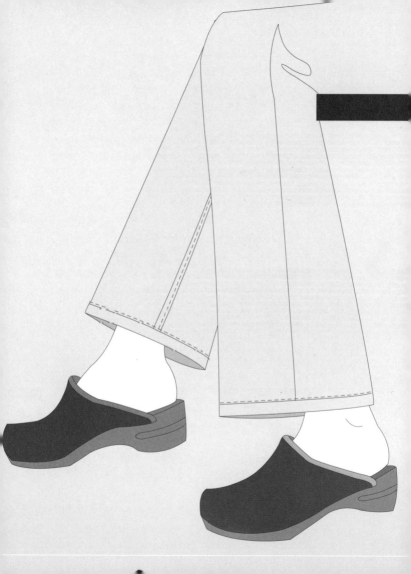

finding a sole mate

Finding mates who are as down-to-earth as you are, are true to themselves, and have a distinctly mellow vibe is important. A Clog girl is never happy with someone who is disingenuous. A natural flow of loving feeling to and from your mate is essential, rather than any wild proclamations of love or, on the contrary, contentious lovers' spats. Consistency and smoothness is the key here.

invoking your inner stiletto

Pulling your hair back in a tight high pony and donning some turquoise chandelier earrings can be a great way to uncover a bit of Inner Stiletto. A bracelet of Japanese redwood, perhaps? Ah, yes.

GETTING A LEG UP

No matter what your Shoe sign, putting your delicate foot into a sumptuous stocking (knee- or thigh-high) can bring a pinch of stiletto to any ensemble. Try fishnets in black or deep eggplant or herringbone cutwork patterns, jacquards or lace, crocheted or ribbed textures, sensual and plush all-cashmere.

retro basketball

Quiet and shy, you are a real dreamer. Creatively blessed, you can just look at a piece of paper and an amazing design will practically appear. You love to read avant-garde glossy magazines, fascinated with the layout, graphics, and pictures, and you have a very defined and particular aesthetic when it comes to your own work. You probably went to a small liberal arts college where you majored in fine arts. You are not a huge socializer, but because you are always one of the coolest cats of the bunch, you are frequently invited to the hottest events. Quiet and a bit indrawn, you can be very shy, but when you look out from those long lashes, you treat others to a kind and inquisitive attention.

completing the look

Definitely an individual, you look best in jeans by an up-and-coming edgy designer, preferably that drag a bit on the ground for a cool ragged-edge effect and a vintage blazer, distressed and a little ripped up, over a custom tee, all in dark hues of black, eggplant, purple, or olive. Your hair is cut in fringy bangs, which cover your eyes a bit, and makeup is minimalist but dramatic — kohl eyeliner, lots of mascara, pale complexion, and a hint of light pink lip gloss all work well to keep the cool effects going.

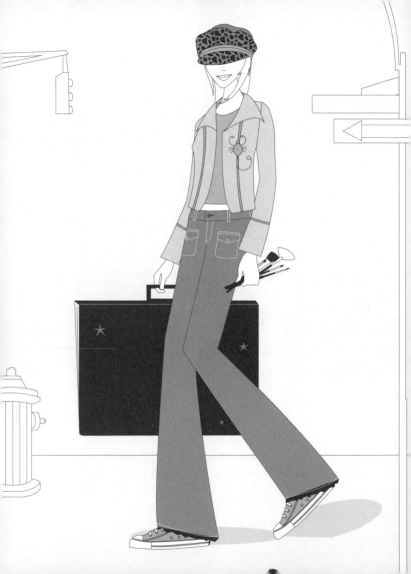

Your dreamy creativeness means that a career in fine art or high fashion suits you well. Though your behind-the-scenes aesthetic make an important impression on the world at large, you yourself are rarely seen in the public eye, choosing to pursue your calling in the background, where your ideas can flourish.

finding a sole mate

Your mates have got to be independent thinkers, a little punky, with an appreciation for the Ramones. Their aesthetics have got to cross over into yours and even match at times in order for you to groove together. You shouldn't even entertain the idea of someone in the business world, instead going for the bassist in the latest electroclash band, graphic designer, or even journalist (though not one in the immediate media glare). A sense of humor is important, for you can tend to be a little melancholy. A partner who can gently lift you with a little joke or two is always beneficial for you.

invoking your inner stiletto

Slashing a deep *V* in that vintage tee of yours and donning a dark maroon nail polish with a subtle sparkle are both nice ways to let your inner stiletto really shine.

on-the-go

One word: *active*. In whatever they do, be it
athletic endeavors, purposeful walking to and from
work, or nights out, these ladies approach
life with determination and zeal. They are health
conscious — life for them always includes
a walk across town or a daily run. They like to
know they are covering ground, even if it
is only to the grocery store and back. Extremely
independent, they tend to have love affairs based
on mutual admiration and fun activities.

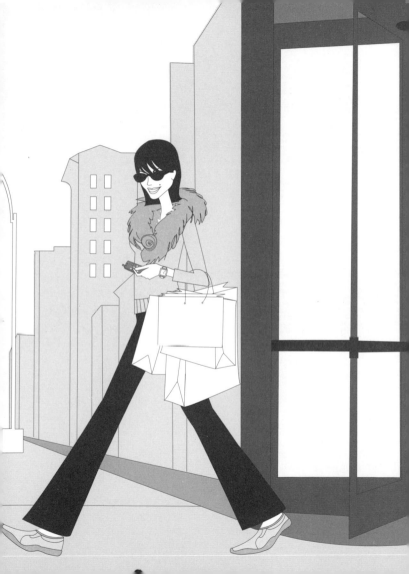

loafer

From the classic penny loafer to the modified modern loafer, loafers signify an American ease, classic styling, and practicality that always envelop the girl who wears them. Whether you're donning a cordovan classic or a molded rubber-heel Italian version, most of you are the essence of common sense. Speedily working things to a satisfying conclusion, you are not afraid to get right into the mix of whatever is going on, be it a business deal or family spat. You lend a mix of good cheer and humor, a down-to-earth perspective, and a commitment to a resolution that suits everyone involved. You are a great best friend to have, a wise counselor who is always up for a bit of fun and is energetic about helping solve your pals' problems just as fast as you solve your own.

completing the look

Make sure you have a fine-weave thin dress sock to wear with your loafer, whatever type it may be. Pants in a solid color, usually black, that are neat, creased, and have a slim-tailored fit and a bit of stretch for easy movement are key. For maximum loafer effect, pants should hang with a slight fold below the ankle, just covering the middle of the shoe nicely. A crisp blouse, with just a bit of starch, in an eggshell blue or white is an appropriate pairing, a slim jacket for day, and for evening a silk cardigan sweater in black work well

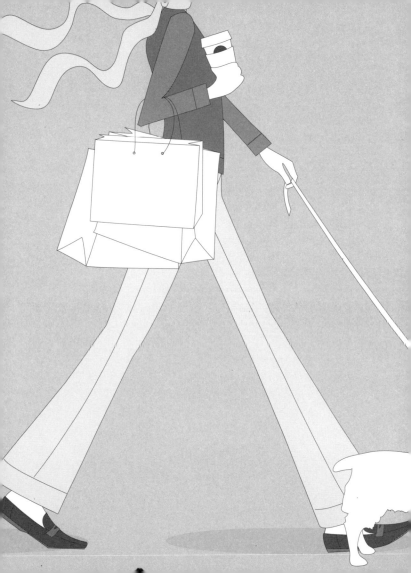

with the pants. If a skirt is desired, try pleated, just above the knee, and a solid-color opaque tight. Hair is neat, a short bob tucked behind the ears or neatly back in a ponytail where nary a wisp escapes. Makeup is a touch of a rosy blush, mascara, and a light pink gloss.

work it, girl

Honestly, if you're a Loafer girl, you are going to do well anywhere you land. Try for a place where your hard work will have a high payoff — an investment bank or a nonprofit you really believe in, because any organization that is lucky to have you will benefit from your enormous drive, diplomacy, and ever-positive willingness to get the job done.

finding a sole mate

You want someone who is just as adept at navigating the world as you are, but it's good if your mates have a knack for silliness as well. This way, they can always be counted on for a bit of fun when you are in the thick of things — an important way for some of your intensity to lessen. Consistency and sense of purpose are key — a mate who knows what life is all about, beyond work and getting things done.

invoking your inner stiletto

How about some thong underwear of a rich, handmade lace? You won't be able to wait to get into your own pants.

sneaker

The Sneaker girl is all about cool, but very accessible cool. Normally seen dashing about town, you always know the coolest music and films. You are quick on your feet and witty, often peppering your conversation with a bit of ironic or sarcastic humor just for effect. And then you're gone just as fast as you arrived.

completing the look

Try flared-leg fine-wale cords in solid bold colors: pumpkin, eggplant, hunter green, or black. A vintage or customized tee under a long-sleeved button-down also of vintage descent completes the look. Hair should be totally natural in whatever form it may take — short spiky and a bit punky, or long and curly. Only makeup that can be applied while in dashing mode will do — lip gloss from a tube, tinted moisturizer with sunscreen, and mascara usually work well. Accoutrements are more often something handmade and rustic — a rope necklace with handmade bead, a sturdy backpack or messenger bag in a bright color that is a bit distressed from constant use.

work it, girl

You have got to be producing something to be happy: film, music, cool lifestyle magazine — whatever it is, it's got to be hipster and zippy. Constant motion is the only state you'll be happy in, so find a place that requires much of you in the

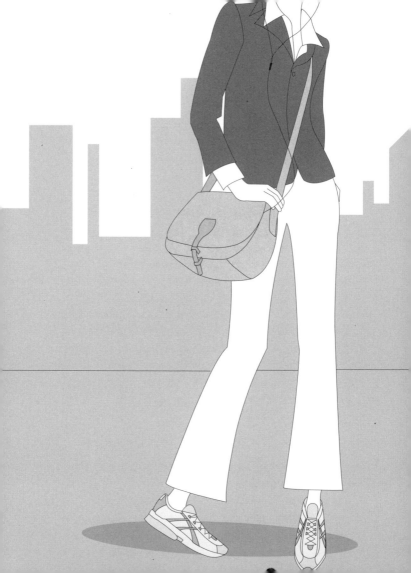

way of shepherding ideas, film canisters, edits, or photography from one place to another, along with your expertise in behind-the-scenes running.

You want someone who will go skateboarding and exploring with you, just as easily as hanging at home on a Saturday afternoon, chilling and listening to the latest French house CD. Your mates have got to be flexible, fun, and actually get your ironic remarks. A little bit of a thick skin helps so that they never get hurt by your ironies, but not too thick. They've got to be able to open up emotionally and listen to your dreams and desires just as well. It's important for a Sneaker girl to feel she always has a place of safe, sweet loving with her mate where she can really open up and lose her freneticism.

invoking your inner stiletto

Showing off your creamy shoulders can be a nice touch. Toss off the layered look and instead try a light pink tank of mercerized cotton with lacy trim to pair with your cords. And some dangly earrings. Voilà!

running shoe

You are recognizable by your very purposeful walk. Outwardly friendly yet also brusque and businesslike, you seem to be extremely buoyant and at the same time very directed in all of your goings to and fro.

Whether you're getting your business-school degree or just going to work out, you are streaming through life with a walk that is grounded. You usually believe that there is nothing in life a little determination and hard work won't solve. Through this lens you view most of life's situations, which can be both extraordinarily uplifting and frustrating to those around you, as you can dole out tactical support with the best of them but can't really understand why someone would ever need an extended crying jag.

completing the look

Complete the look with a pair of khakis and a high-quality cotton tee. You don't want anything to interfere with your freedom of movement or air of purposefulness. To appear neat, approachable, and hardworking at all times, your hair is either in a bob or a neat ponytail; either way it is all one length — no layers.

Wear your college ring and a string of pearls. Because you wear pretty serious running shoes, it always seems like you are leaning in a little bit, like a runner getting ready for a sprint. And in some ways you are, since you are always getting ready for the next challenge life is handing you. Light

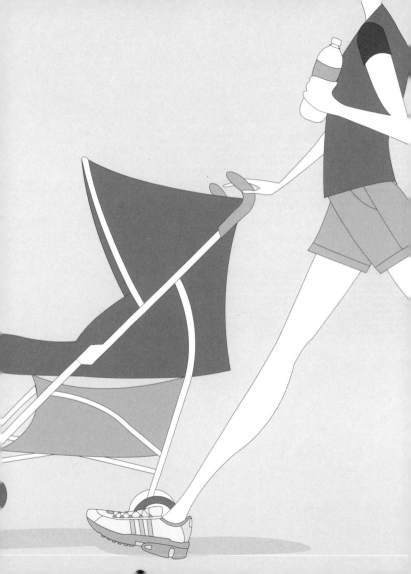

pink lip gloss and a touch of rosy blush complete your energetic look.

work it, girl

If you are not a world-class athlete yourself, you are running a global, market-making corporation.

finding a sole mate

You'll easily find your Sole Mate while you are out running one day. Your mate will respond to your sense of purpose and your natural cheery demeanor. You need someone who will be able to run the marathons of life with you, a cheerleader and a steady confidant.

invoking your inner stiletto

A nice way to do this is slowing your run all the way down to a walk. Get into the present moment and make each step a slow, gliding, feminine, seductive movement.

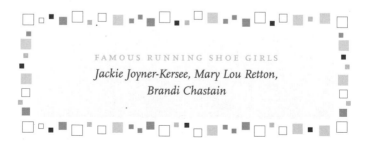

FAMOUS RUNNING SHOE GIRLS
Jackie Joyner-Kersee, Mary Lou Retton,
Brandi Chastain

designer bowling shoe

You've got a penchant for strenuous tasks. Running and climbing, you like to tackle the impossible project, the immovable object, and always root for the underdog. An asset to everyone, you'll fight like the dickens for them or their cause. Scrappy and resourceful, you are the girl I'd like to have around if I suddenly found myself in a dangerous situation. You're prone to action, with thinking on your feet your specialty. Your sense of humor is renowned; you find the absurd in everyday life and laugh heartily, often roping everyone around you in on the joke.

completing the look

Durable jeans or cords in solid black, burnt orange, or hunter green that have been worn in are a great choice if you're a DBS girl. Since movement is a constant with you, try easy flexible pieces that are uncomplicated and coordinated enough to wear layered, like long- and short-sleeved tees, an occasional sweater turtleneck, and the ever-present tank in a feminine cut with some girly accoutrement. Hair is either short and choppy or swept up in a messy bun, and mascara, eyeliner, and lipstick are a must — they give you an easy lift throughout your hectic day. Jewelry is always a piece or two from your travels — both exotic and a conversation starter. If you've got to dress it up a bit, try a neatly tailored jacket in a fine cotton twill.

You've got to be constantly engaged in your work and idealistically married to it. Good matches are working as a documentary film producer or production assistant, at a nonprofit that does community outreach in underprivileged neighborhoods, or fundraising for one of these. Any organization you choose will benefit from your hard-driving yet fun work ethic and be moved forward by your idealism.

finding a sole mate

You need mates who are comfortable in everyday chaos and don't mind the underdog (or various other animals) being brought home every once in a while for refuge. They've got to be interested in the same causes you are or at least have a deep appreciation for them. Humor is key, as everyday laughter is a must for you.

invoking your inner stiletto

A lacy, sheer black tank under an eggplant purple velvet jacket is always a nice change. Now try a pair of slim, pegged jeans instead of cords, and you are well on your way!

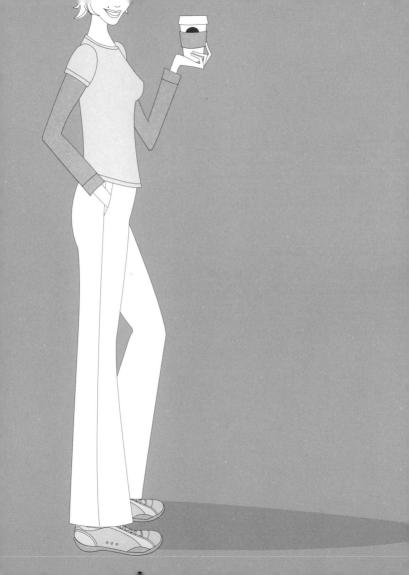

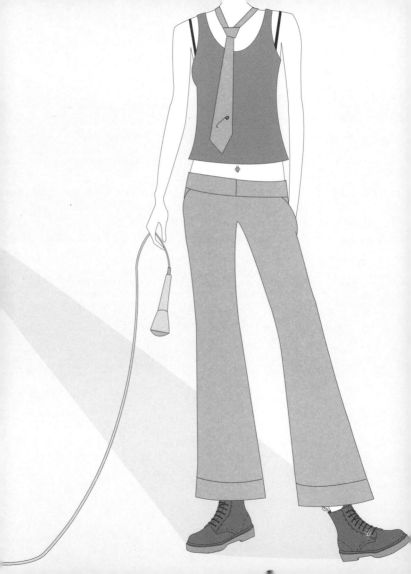

workingman's boot

You may be kicking someone's ass at the moment, metaphorically, of course. At the very least, you are probably standing up for yourself, reading someone the riot act, or kicking in the fender of the taxi that just tried to overcharge you.

Your inner spirit is sometimes more in sync with volcanoes than any other type of shoe girl. You are prone to explosion, but this is good, because you assist society and culture by constantly agitating and forcing people to reexamine their own behavior. We dearly need you to keep things lively — that's for sure.

A Workingman's Boot girl customarily believes that agitation is the spice of life. Most happy when things are really cooking, swinging, and generally happening, you often find yourself in the middle of cultural movements, mosh pits, and PTA uprisings. Fortunately, your sense of fear is minimal, and your ease in these situations is high. Not always the leader of these movements, you are sometimes the volatile sidekick, inspiring everyone to take action with your rousing words that follow (or occur during) the headliner's speech. To be comfortable with you is to be comfortable with the fact that any given situation is rich ground for dissent.

It is important for you to be fully expressed in your wardrobe, hair, and makeup. Hair looks great spiky, and color is an important element for a WB girl. Body art usually figures prominently; it is important for you to feel that your body is a true expression of your beliefs and causes. Try looks that allow for martial art kicks when needed — baggy black parachute pants, a pleated mini with distressed black tights, and a leather coat so that you can feel protected. If you are of the fully butching-it variety, a white tee, denim overalls, and a large swagger help you feel fully in your Workingman's Boot element.

While a coffeehouse may seem like an odd place for you to land, it is often a good place for you. You have free java to keep you wired, an ear to a lot of different movements in the community, and a flexible work schedule, which is great since going to see bands play in the evening is a major part of your happiness. That is, if you're not playing in the band, which is another great occupation for you. Getting your screeching guitar and heavy drum on in a serious downtown garage rock band or fronting the latest angry female hit machine is a wonderful way for you to express yourself — and support yourself, to boot.

Loyalty is the No. 1 recommended trait for you to feel happy and secure in a relationship. Because you find yourself in a higher number than average of altercations, physical strength is another, as you want to know that when looking out for your back, your mate can also go to bat for you in a pinch. An exception to this is the butch lady. You, on the contrary, are better matched with someone petite, feminine, and in a flouncy miniskirt.

invoking your inner stiletto

A wonderful way to up the ante is by wearing the black pants a little tighter and outlining the delicious pear that you are. You didn't know you were a sweet pear? Oh *yes*, you are.

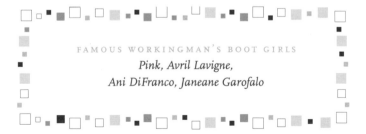

FAMOUS WORKINGMAN'S BOOT GIRLS
*Pink, Avril Lavigne,
Ani DiFranco, Janeane Garofalo*

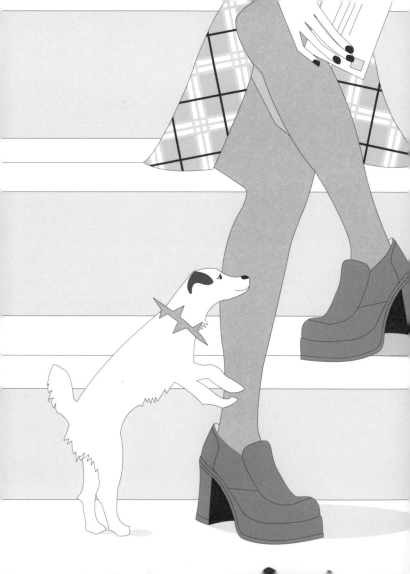

clunky chunky-heel loafer

The Clunky Chunky-Heel Loafer girl plays an important role in our society. You are the unformed thinker in the midst of putting together your beliefs. You are both an examining observer of what goes on around you and an active participant. Usually young, high school, college, or just post, you hang around with your girlfriends in large packs. A bit of the Goth girl in your soul, you are constantly weighing what people actually say and do against conventional wisdom. A bit fierce and possessing what can seem like a rather distant or cold disposition, at the heart of the matter you're a sweet, almost grown-up girl, trying to reconcile your emotions and feelings with the outside world.

completing the look

Try a pleated skirt with tights, wool sweater, and a parka, and for dress-up, tailored shiny pants and a neat blouse. Hair thrown up into a messy bun is cute or maybe short with a bit of punkiness to it. Multiple ear piercings help establish the independent spirit look, along with the odd tattoo, usually of a spiritual nature. Eye makeup is a must, in dark colors, and always mascara.

work it, girl

You need a flexible schedule and an occupation that allows for reading on the job. A waitress or coffee slinger at a small bistro or coffeehouse usually fills the bill. Being around other thinkers doesn't hurt either, so assisting a professor can be a good fit (but only if the professor is respectful and bereft of academic snobbery).

finding a sole mate

You need a mate who can truly be a friend first, one who prizes your independent spirit and is as interested in discovering the world as you are. Your mate has got to like music and accompany you to the many indie bands you like to go see. Well read and sweet, maybe even a little shy, this someone is quietly individualistic and totally taken with you.

invoking your inner stiletto

Highlight your sexy neck by working your hair into a sleek bun or wet-gelling it back close to the head, if it's short. Add a pair of chandelier earrings to heighten the effect, and you're there.

hiking boot

You are intrepid. You have no problem hiking over a mountain, stream, glacier, or other natural creation. You move with assuredness through life, often intuiting what the next right step is before you make it. After years of adventures, you've learned to trust yourself, and your air of quiet confidence is unshakable. Having faced many of nature's absurdities, you've got a hilarious sense of humor and a built-in hardiness that can withstand even the most grueling of conditions. But make no mistake, you also possess a very feminine allure, that of the woman-adventurer, a free spirit who knows the value of her own footstep.

completing the look

Get into warm, flexible fleece pants, treated with waterproofing, that tuck easily into your boots or adjust with a pulley. Zip-up fleeces and turtlenecks in bright colors are only one of the many layers that are advantageous for you to wear. Hair is either cropped short or long and tied back in a ponytail. Makeup tends to be a waterproof sunscreen of high SPF, lip protectant, and a natural glowing radiance that comes from being active and outdoors. You may have the odd bit of whimsy, a fun necklace from one of the many tribes you've met, a charm on your fleece zipper from home, even a tattoo or two.

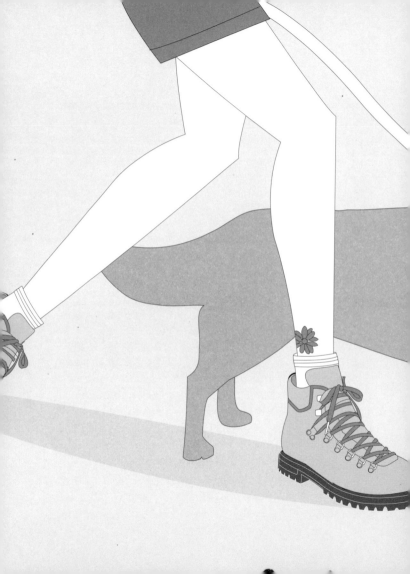

You've got to be outside and using your body and hands to be happy. Working as a biologist in the field, an anthropologist studying tribal cultures, an archaeologist digging up the latest Egyptian tomb, a navigator of snow caves, or a *National Geographic* producer are all excellent matches for you.

finding a sole mate

It's best if your mate is in the same field as you so that coordinating together time is a minimum hassle. Plus, it's good for you to work side by side with your mate; there's nothing better for your spirit than to be in your element and have the one you love along for the ride. Your mate's got to be able to roll with the punches nature throws at you two together and laugh along with you just as heartily.

invoking your inner stiletto

Replace your laces with wide pink satin ribbons and tie them in a large floppy bow. The wideness of the ribbon will ensure that they last through your next jungle adventure, and the pink will remind you of your feminine side as you conquer the elements.

cowboy boot

You could be an actual cowgirl on the prairie or a city girl with a cowgirl heart. Either way, you've got a zing about you, a little extra panache that comes from inherent confidence. You probably know how to rope a steer or head up a multimillion-dollar film. With an intensity that runs deep, your penetrating eyes get to the bottom of things, even in the most casual conversation.

completing the look

The No. 1 wardrobe essential for you should be jeans. Slim-fitting, to the waist, dark or faded, and easy to move in. A long, flowing skirt is a close second. For the city girl, a bit of glitz on the top is always a perfect complement: maybe a customized tee with lacy accoutrement. For the girl on the range, a typical cowboy shirt works well, with some feminine braiding. Hair in a ponytail is helpful, even if it is wisping out just a bit, since you could be herding cattle or engineering a movie shoot, but it's better that it not get in the way of the major project at hand.

work it, girl

Straight-shooting work is best. A Cowboy Boot girl should not be assigned any extraneous tasks, only projects that let you get your hands dirty, roll up your sleeves, and start kicking. Whether film director or chef or ranch owner, all CB

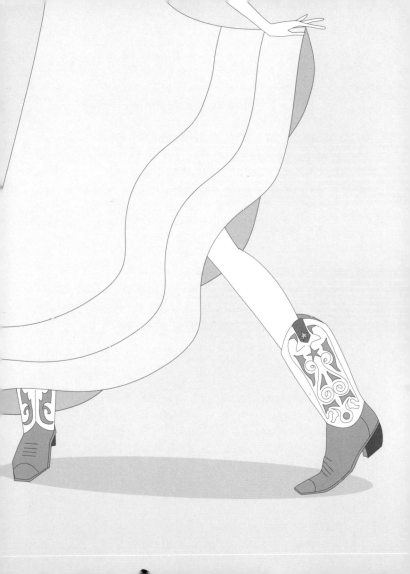

girls have one thing in common workwise, and that is you like getting the job done.

finding a sole mate

Interestingly, you are actually rather private. A good Sole Mate match for you is someone who is a bit quiet when it comes to matters of the heart, who will appreciate you for your energy but not be overly demonstrative. It is imperative that your mate be a solid partner and a gentle comfort and support to you when your hard-drivin' day is done.

invoking your inner stiletto

Convert the jeans into some hip-hugging, low-riding stretchy numbers and show off a little bit of your luscious curves, lower back, and a peek of your panties. Cute!

VINTAGE

Miss Meghan loves to get her hands on a good vintage find. A vintage shoe is a worldly accessory, one that walked miles and lived another life before finding its way to you. The drawback, of course, is that aged heel — a bit dry with a tendency to crack or split, sometimes at very inopportune times. (Note to self: Do not wear vintage stilettos when accepting your Oscar.)

knee-high boot with low heel

As on-the-go as all the other girls, you are very dedicated to looking sleek as you zoom from place to place. You favor a black boot, with a molded rubber or stacked wood heel, made from a fine leather. The knee high boot with low heel gives you added flair as you have a tendency to wear it with skirts, thus giving a bit of a sassy vibe to your comings and goings. You are a fount of common sense, always at the ready with a hearty laugh or a bit of practical advice. You know how to change a tire on a car, but if you're with a man, you'll let him do it just to make him feel like a hero.

completing the look

For your days zipping about town, try bootleg slim-fit jeans with a solid color tee and a corduroy jacket. For evening events, a just-below-the-knee A-line skirt works well with a slim turtle-neck sweater — thick-ply cashmere, of course, or a pretty embroidered tank and a denim jacket. Makeup is simple and clean — no fuss, lip gloss, sheer color on the cheeks, and a bit of mascara; in the evenings, a tiny hint of sparkle around the eyes brings out your playfulness. Jewelry is classic: pearl or diamond studs.

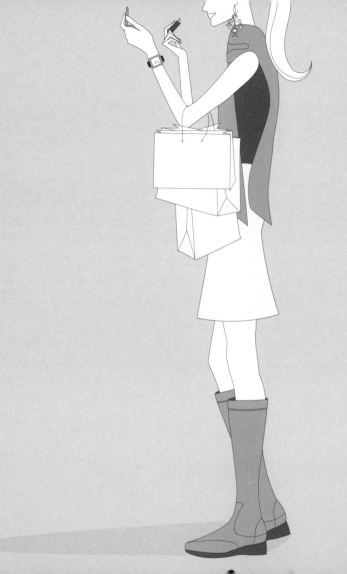

You've got to be in an artistic pursuit to be happy. Whether this means you are a writer, visual artist, sculptor, or musician, or work for any of the above, you've got to have your hand in some creative place to feel fully alive.

finding a sole mate

Your mates have got to have a jolly side to them. A mate who is too buttoned up will simply not work with you, because for all your practicality, you like to have a lot of fun in everyday life. A mate with solid middle-class values and a steady job is always beneficial since your income might be a bit chaotic.

invoking your inner stiletto

I want to see some sexy crocheted tights in a dark purple under your A-line skirt. Just a peek of the knee in these, and you'll be inciting riots. In a good way.

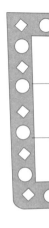

towering heights

Towering Heights Girls love their heels.
They adore the click of their sound on
the pavement, the arch they create in their foot,
the slight sway they create in their walk, the
lengthening of the leg, the slimming of
the silhouette, the headiness of the view from up
there. These ladies love their air a little thinner.
On the whole, they tend to be a bit more involved
in their appearance and are always very
interested in presenting a carefully prepared
persona. They are more given to passionate
love affairs and fall in love easily. And they, more
than the other fundamental shoe girls, like
to dress up on an everyday basis.

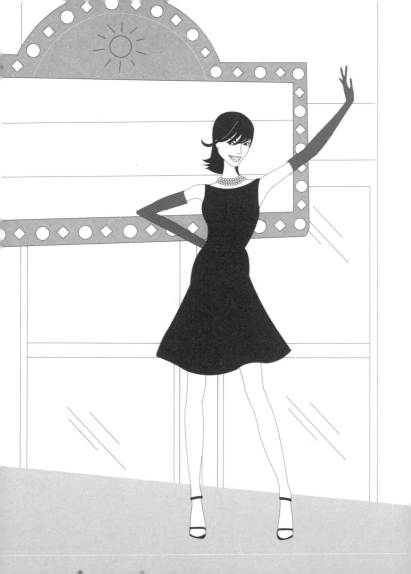

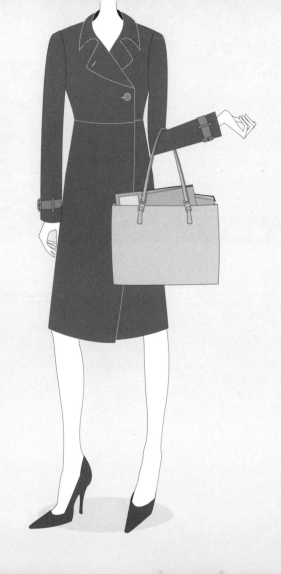

classic conservative pump

You may be diligently scanning the *Financial Times* and *Wall Street Journal* on your way to work at an investment bank, an accounting firm, or a law firm. You most likely have a cup of coffee in one hand, the paper in another, and an overstuffed laptop bag. Appearing a bit discombobulated, you are actually simultaneously reading the paper, scanning your text messages, drinking your coffee, and jotting a note for your morning meeting in your PDA.

You are a most loyal friend, unflagging in your ability to show up for any event, any time of day, always available for a quick joke and a laugh. Extraordinarily good-natured and extremely resilient, you've got a man's *fraternité* and affability, making you a most valued friend since you are always so easygoing. Smart as a whip, you can rattle off stock indexes as easily as the latest baseball scores without missing a beat. You can work until 4 A.M., be in the office at 8 A.M., and still make it to your best friend's birthday party that evening with a smile on your face and the perfect present in your hands.

Your values are basic: work hard, get paid well, use your brain, value your family and friends, and give back. You are not overly cheery in bad situations, but rather rock solid and consistently pleasant.

Five or six interchangeable navy and black suits, one with a pinstripe (plus a few light-khaki linen ones thrown in for summer), are neat, easy looks for you. Because ease of movement is essential, wearing pants with your jackets and a simple blouse or a fine-weave cashmere sweater work best. Jewelry is minimal — a pair of pearls or diamond studs, a school ring, and a necklace from your sweet sixteen work. Best if your hair is kept back during the workday and out of fussing range. Lip gloss is all you need — your complexion is usually very good and always has a natural bit of rosy glow.

work it, girl

A law firm, accounting firm, or investment bank are good choices, that is, if you are not president of your own media company or a CEO already. You worked your tail off in school, Ivy League, summa cum laude, and were involved in multiple extracurricular clubs, including fundraising and tutoring for underprivileged children.

finding a sole mate

You need the same great qualities that make you a standout: constant, resilient, good-natured, and fun. Fortunately, you assume this is what everyone is like and because you never lower your standards, you've always got an adoring mate and loads of friends.

Don a few pieces of pink lacy French lingerie before you don your suit and pair it with a pink button-down instead of your usual white. With just one too many buttons undone, you are very subtly but deliberately invoking a bit of your Inner Stiletto.

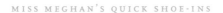

MISS MEGHAN'S QUICK SHOE-INS

Wondering what to wear
for that all-important occasion?

JOB INTERVIEW WITH UBER-CREATIVE/HIGH-FASHION
CORPORATION: *designer stiletto*

FIRST DATE: *ballet flat in soft pink*

BREAKING UP WITH BOYFRIEND: *black, extremely*
thin-heeled stiletto (so you can walk away with studied,
sexy determination, leaving him salivating in your wake)

THIRD DATE WITH POTENTIAL SOLE MATE:
kitten heel or stiletto, any style or color

SHOPPING AND LUNCHING WITH GIRLFRIENDS:
flat mule or knee-high boot with high heel

t-strap

Ta-daaaa! A T-Strap girl always arrives with a bit of a splash. You are either in your latest Broadway musical or just taking the everyday office water-cooler talk up a notch. Always a bit peppier than those around you, you have a penchant for launching into a show tune, which has everyone else laughing and singing along. If they don't know the words, you'll give a quick, good-natured lesson. Others can't really help but be infected by your natural gutsiness and Betty Boop–like cuteness. You often look like you stepped off the set of a '40s movie, steno in hand.

completing the look

T-Strap girls always look good in a slim, structured skirt and a neatly tucked-in cotton blouse for a daytime office gig. In the evening, a pair of fishnets adds a bit of theatricality and fun, paired with a slim skirt and simple boatneck top in black jersey for ease of movement.

work it, girl

If you are not actually living in your T-straps for your latest gig on Broadway, you do best in an office where you can showcase your natural showwomanship and be appreciated for your virtues. A film company is always a good match, and any studio would be lucky to have you — you can easily

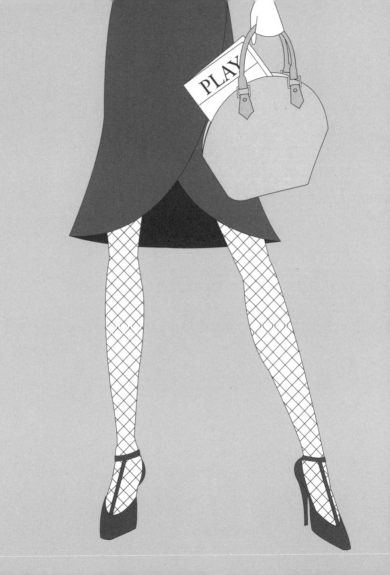

manage a chaotic environment with your good nature and penchant for song. Your unique ability to manage up (with little or no knowledge on the part of those being managed) always adds a sweet hum to any environment, turning any place you land into a well-oiled machine.

finding a sole mate

This lady needs a song mate, one who will whistle a tune from *42nd Street* under his breath and look quizzically up at you, daring you to name the tune on the spot. Your playfulness needs to be matched in pure fun — a bump on a log or shrinking violet is not for you.

invoking your inner stiletto

A draped top that shows off your shoulders is a great way to show off some sacred flesh. Just lovely.

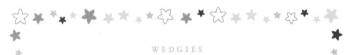

WEDGIES

Wedge heels are a wonderful invention. They give you height and often are more cushy and comfortable than a sharp stiletto heel. They also add a bit of 1940s vintage glamour to any look.

open toe

Getting on your boyfriend's Vespa just outside a hip café in the coolest part of town, you are averse to a helmet since it will mess with your carefully coiffed '40s updo with cute bangs. You might be zipping off to a gig where a mix of vintage jazz and modern doo-wop is the main attraction. Or maybe you are in your 1965 Cadillac convertible on your way to the flea market. Wherever you are off to, you usually make a sassy entrance with your shiny open-toe heels that tilt you just a little forward, put an extra zing in your walk, and give onlookers a tiny peek of the toe cleavage.

completing the look

Skirts, mostly in the "New Look" style, full and waist-accentuating, show off your natural flair. Shirtwaists should figure prominently, veering toward a more classic '60s silhouette. If you're a curvaceous gal, you should accentuate your figure. If you're not entirely buxom, accenting the curviest parts of your body with a little dart and a tuck is perfect. With jeans, the bottoms should be rolled up, shirt elegantly tied around your waist. Lipstick should always be in a darker shade of red or violet and always be applied. (An Open-Toe Shoe girl with naked lips is not recommended.)

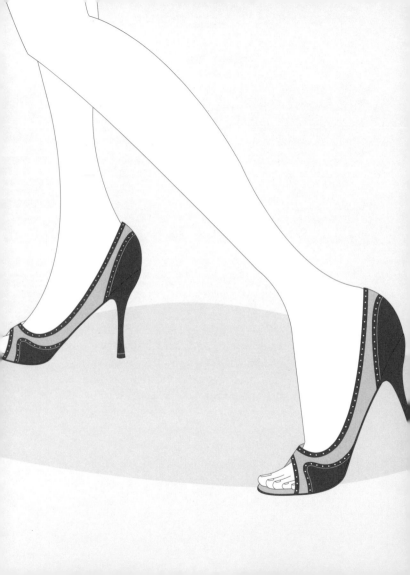

As an Open-Toe girl, you do best in an extremely detail-oriented and artistic career. Naturally very discerning about your occupation, careers as a vintage eyeglass or art restorer, upholsterer, or wallpaper designer are all good matches for you. Since you are extremely practical in all matters of business, you excel at owning your own business and are often renowned in your aesthetic circles for your work.

finding a sole mate

You will do well with mates who are appreciative of the fine arts. They've got to be able to hang at a museum as well as the local jazz bar. You also work well with mates who are good with their hands: carpenters, wrought-iron workers, and sculptors are good matches for you.

invoking your inner stiletto

A silk halter top shows off your gorgeous arms and shoulders. Make sure the halter ties in a cheeky little bow at the back of the neck for extra Stiletto.

knee-high boot with high heel

A Knee-High Boot with High-Heel girl is most likely committed to the life of the bourgeoisie; middle-class values to you are the true essence of life. Education is highly prized, and you are well read, kind to all you encounter, a solid citizen, and a rock-solid foundation to your family and friends. Your sense of humor is unflappable; you value hard work and believe in regular holidays and the importance of being neatly turned out at all times. You have three or four pairs of black high-heel knee-high boots that you get cleaned, resoled, and repaired every spring. When one pair finally reaches the end of its sometimes fifteen-year run, you carefully hit the first fall sale to replace it.

completing the look

You favor classic looks — and you should. Your shoes reveal your inherent classic taste in everything from music to furniture, and your looks are often representative of that as well. Tailored slacks with a merino wool tiny cabled twin set in a bright color and your hair neatly arranged in a bob or pulled pack in a neat ponytail are good looks for you. For evening, a long skirt with a slit in front up to the knee, showing off your boots, paired with a silk top in a jewel tone or evening jacket works best.

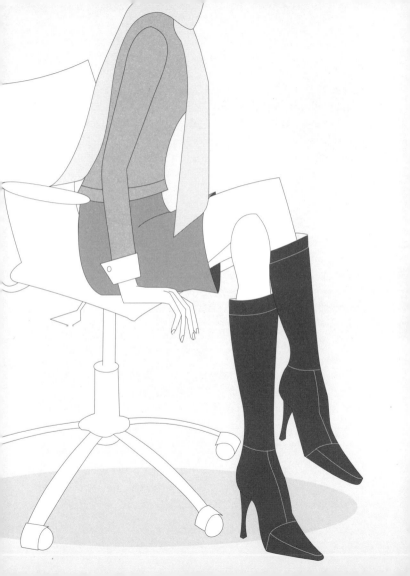

You work well in professions that are structured and perceived as steady and prestigious. Banking is a good fit for you, though most likely you'll fit better in the marketing department than on a trading floor. You're the one who communicates the best with senior management and CEOs; as a consequence, you usually rise to a top position at whatever firm you land at.

finding a sole mate

Trusty is the No. 1 trait you should look for in a mate. Your heart needs to know your mate is always there for you through the good and the bad, for celebrating the joys of life with you and being a solid presence in your life. Consistency is a key trait, and you deserve a mate with this quality for it is one of your own shining virtues.

invoking your inner stiletto

Try a boot with a wild design, one with unusual textures like python or snake or cow stomach — or even one with bold colored patterns and cutwork — scalloped edging, contrasting stitching, or metallic heels. Yeah, baby!

ankle boot with high heel

You may be stepping out of a sleek black hired car in the city or lunching at a top restaurant. You are definitely both accustomed to luxury and fully in the mix of the latest social goings-on. You can slice and dice a business deal in two shakes of your pony-skin bag and at the same time negotiate your two-year-old and five-year-old's spat of the moment with an earthy intuition. You are matter-of-fact feminine, at ease in your skin and your abilities.

completing the look

Recommended gear for this girl are tight-fitting jeans and a slim cashmere sweater for day, and for evening, jeans or slim-fitting satin pants paired with a sparkly top. Your hair is usually best worn down and framing the face, with neutral makeup; a mauve-tinted lipstick or even a neutral lip work well for you. This combination of body-hugging clothes and careful makeup gives you an added edge — you are no doubt one of the most feminine creatures others have ever encountered; yet you are no-nonsense and down-to-earth at the same time.

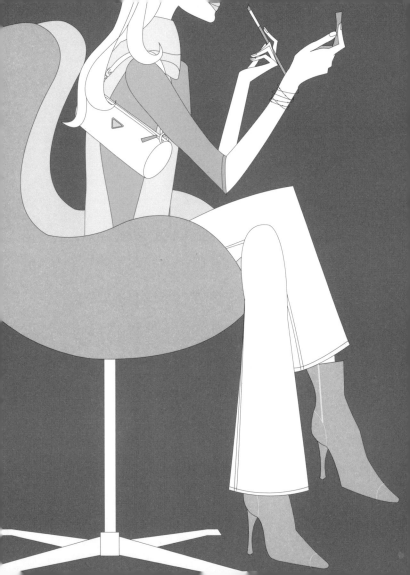

You have a special talent for getting things done in a very frank and open way. You are just as straightforward in any kind of business dealing and are always in the mood to strike a bargain. For this reason, you are happiest in professions that require a lot of wheeling and dealing and relationship skills. Real estate is an excellent choice for you, as well as owning a modeling agency, construction company, general contracting company, or even a sports team.

finding a sole mate

You need a mate who will take care of you, who will navigate the city streets to make sure you don't snag your heel in a hole or get thrown off balance. Your mate has to like luxury and spoil you with all the trappings a woman like you desires; this will be rewarded by a happy woman, as devoted and loyal as a lioness toward her cubs.

invoking your inner stiletto

Try some just-kissed red lipstick. For a beautiful highlight to one of your loveliest assets, go for the shade your lips would be had you just engaged in a lusty makeout session.

mule with high heel

You are most often found in a sunny climate, preferring the summer season to all others. Most likely, you've just served a guest a fruity pink drink from a pink tray and are now sitting down next to your guest, poolside, with a copy of *Cosmopolitan* in your hand, just for fun. More often than not, you are the hostess of whatever summertime poolside gathering all your girlfriends are attending, whether it be a just-for-two spa lunch or a full-on barbecue.

completing the look

Pink and lime-green capri pants in a Palm Beach print, paired with a white shirtwaist. Slim, black, cotton capri pants are a close second, paired with a red-and-white-striped boatneck with three-quarter sleeves. In the evening, the capri pant is paired with a taffeta or silk shell and pearls. Hair is in a ponytail, and sunglasses are a must-have accessory, no matter what time of day. Any skirt should be short and straight — no flounces.

work it, girl

You typically excel at any position in the decorative arts. From working in interior design to wardrobe consultation to flower arranging, you add a flair to anything you put your hands on and are most happy when making something more beautiful.

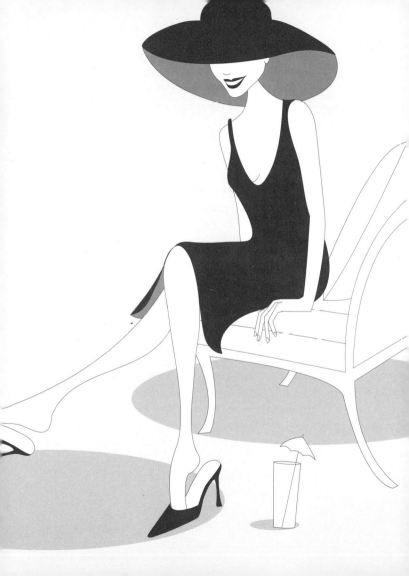

finding a sole mate

Your mate has got to be above average in looks and well groomed. You must be able to link arms with your mate down the street and feel that together, you make a beautiful couple.

invoking your inner stiletto

You've got the height going on. Trying a silk jacquard bustier in a jewel tone of red or deep magenta instead of the taffeta shell for evening is a lovely way to highlight those beautiful neck and shoulders of yours.

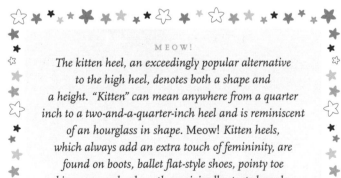

MEOW!

The kitten heel, an exceedingly popular alternative to the high heel, denotes both a shape and a height. "Kitten" can mean anywhere from a quarter inch to a two-and-a-quarter-inch heel and is reminiscent of an hourglass in shape. Meow! Kitten heels, which always add an extra touch of femininity, are found on boots, ballet flat-style shoes, pointy toe skimmers, and, where they originally started, mules. A kitten is an acceptable Miss Meghan– sanctioned alternative to a stiletto any day.

high-heel sandal

The woman who finds herself in high-heel sandals for a majority of her shoe time is a woman who is very confident in her femininity. Toes are most likely always pedicured perfectly in coral or pink. Your ability to balance a cocktail tray, glass of wine, piece of hardware or two, soccer ball, and the odd child or two in both hands, while glowing with feminine wiles, is a testament to your balancing prowess in all matters of life, your determination, and your extremely strong ab muscles. You are a woman who has the very special ability to make things just a little more festive than they were before you arrived, a quality much needed in this world.

completing the look

You look best in very feminine colors and fabrics — light and dark pinks, taffetas, silks, white, corals. Tailored pants, often capri-style to show off the ankle, or very short skirts work well for the High-Heel Sandal girl. Looks are best as simple and classic, not frilly, and always with a distinct accoutrement — a lovely pin, a ribbon or two, a charm bracelet dangling fetchingly from your wrist.

work it, girl

The most important quality for your work is that it actively engage you. Whether you are a mom, an interior designer, a general contractor, a professional organizer, or a real estate

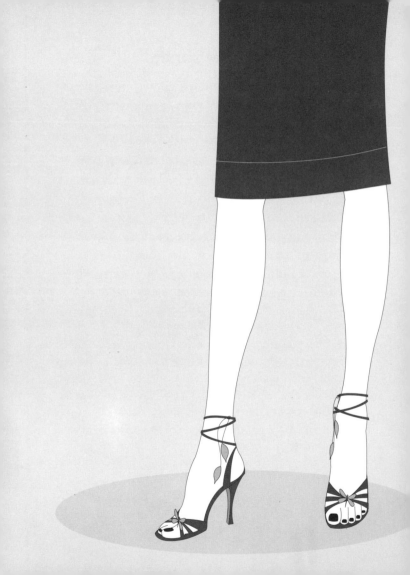

maven, you've got to be consistently moving from one project to the next in order to keep yourself in tip-top shape.

finding a sole mate

You need someone cozy to cozy up to, someone who adores you and appreciates your femininity in every single one of its forms. You like to be taken care of and also like to take care of your mates, spoiling them from time to time with surprise gifts and always lots of love.

invoking your inner stiletto

Already embracing your power of height, go for a sandal with a strap and saucy flower, paired with a short skirt. Lovely.

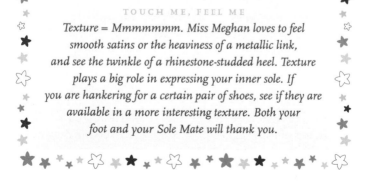

TOUCH ME, FEEL ME

Texture = Mmmmmmm. Miss Meghan loves to feel smooth satins or the heaviness of a metallic link, and see the twinkle of a rhinestone-studded heel. Texture plays a big role in expressing your inner sole. If you are hankering for a certain pair of shoes, see if they are available in a more interesting texture. Both your foot and your Sole Mate will thank you.

designer shoe

The average person might hear you before they actually see you. You are usually an octave louder than the other girls, and moving faster, for that matter, often but a streak on the sidewalk, a whir in your Mercedes. You might just be the one in the car yelling and gesturing at the car in front of you because the driver stopped too quickly.

Constantly on the move, your mantra is action. Typically, you can angle for a bargain faster than one can say "please" and negotiate better than a grizzled CEO. (Designer Shoe girls are good to have on one's side when buying anything from a house to a new wardrobe.) Everyone will be happy (including the opposing party) with the deal you strike. Perfectly manicured, you like things neat, beautiful, and brought to a satisfactory conclusion for all.

Most of you Designer Shoe girls believe that the nice things in life are your right, and you are willing to work for them (even if "work" means looking exceedingly good at society and charity events). You are usually up-front about what you want in friendship, work, or love, a very refreshing trait indeed.

completing the look

Did I mention "designer"? You should find yourself in designer jeans, designer suits, designer nail polish, designer scarves, designer bags, and designer face cream. Especially when you know the designers themselves! Tailored looks —

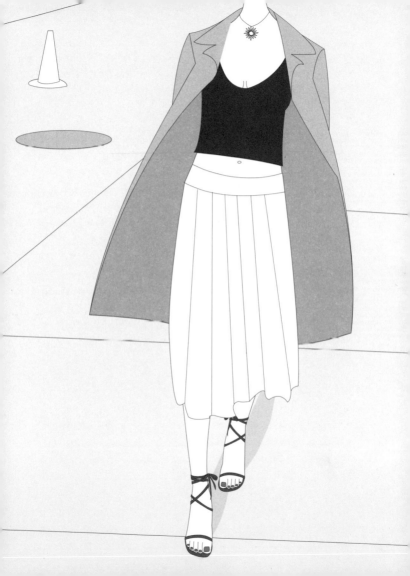

slim jacket and skirt or tailored pants for daytime, and something sparkling and unusual for the evening, be it a dress, a fancy top paired with jeans, or just a bauble in the ear.

work it, girl

An asset to any organization, you get it done in seconds flat, for the lowest price and at the highest standard of luxury. If you are not a high-profile personality yourself, a PR position, captain of a real estate empire, or behind the scenes as a celebrity handler (for a musician, movie star, or fashion designer) are all good fits for you. You are the woman holding the unseen keys to power and prestige.

finding a sole mate

Did I say "prestige"? That would be your sweetie's middle name Your mates must exude it from their pores. You need to be on the arm of someone who's got a commanding presence, enough to match your own.

invoking your inner stiletto

Adding a shoe accoutrement — clip-on jewels, silk flowers, ribbons, or even a very delicate feminine chain around the ankle — is key for you, since you've probably already reached Stiletto heights.

stiletto

You move through the world with an uber-confident horsey walk and are often found on a city street, hailing a cab while talking on your phone. An intriguing mix of traditional and modern, deep down you believe in the fact that men provide and women look good. At the same time, you embrace your raw female power, stepping out smartly, never afraid to state what you want. You are extremely self-possessed and very much your own woman.

completing the look

You work your shoe into most any look with ease, well aware of its leg-lengthening, streamlining advantages. Try tailored jeans and a customized tee on a weekend day or a vampy, '40s-era, black straight-skirted dress for evening cocktails (emphasizing a tiny bit of the S&M properties inherent in a pair of towering black stilettos). At work, an A-line slim-fitting skirt and matching jacket with slim streamlined lapels and neatly tucked-in blouse work well. Makeup is precise and should include a darker shade of lipstick — either red or violet — worn regardless of season or trend. Hair is immaculately trimmed and often tied back in an elegant ponytail or neatly brushed and is always shiny.

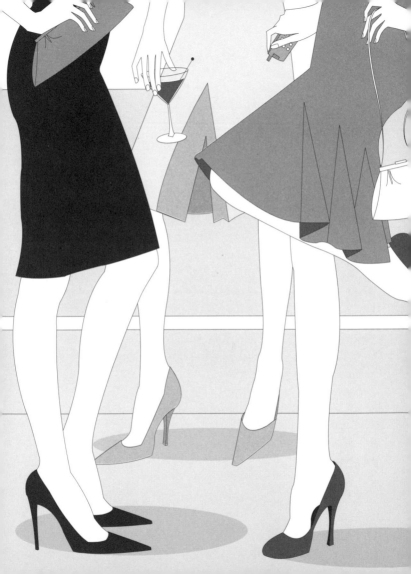

Your natural self-confidence means you'll make a great entertainment executive, performer, owner of a PR firm, or editor in chief at a major fashion magazine. Your shoes establish you as an alpha-female even before you begin to speak. There is no doubt who runs things when you arrive on the scene.

finding a sole mate

Power, elegance, and self-possession. That's really it.

invoking your inner stiletto

Add a red satin ribbon tied in a bow around your neck and see what happens next.

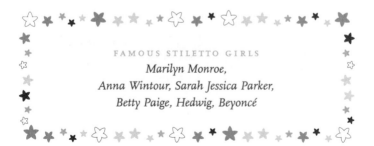

FAMOUS STILETTO GIRLS

Marilyn Monroe,
Anna Wintour, Sarah Jessica Parker,
Betty Paige, Hedwig, Beyoncé

acknowledgments

Thanks, Mom, for always feeding my inner artist; Grandma Helen, for being joyful; Grandma Jane, for graciousness, Aunt Mary, for letting me be the mudge; my dad, for always turning up the hilarity a few notches; my brother, for knowing me; and my entire extended family for their cheerleading.

To my whole team of believers who offered me love, support, advice, and inspiration along the journey of shoe — I love you. Lora & JJ Appleton; Leslie Blanco; Jason Campbell; Tracy Cox; Chef Daniel; Jordan Davis; Mary Donnelly; Rayya Elias; Joe Epstein; Heidi Ewing; Elena Frigeri; my Delta Gamma ladies; Kristin, John & Jack Hall; Amy Holman; Aunt Kit; Jean Loscalzo; Sarah Lukashok; Mama Gena; Raymond McDaniel; Liz McDonald; the folks at Opto Design; Alexandra Rowley; Wendy Shanker; Ann Marie Simonelli; Jason & Randy Sklar; Russell Suggs; and all my sister goddesses.

I'd also like to thank my esteemed agent, Elisabeth Weed; my brilliant editrixes, Mikyla Bruder & Lisa Campbell; my copy editors, Jan Hughes, Doug Ogan, and Susan Lake; and Sydney VanDyke for her gorgeous illustrations. Kisses.